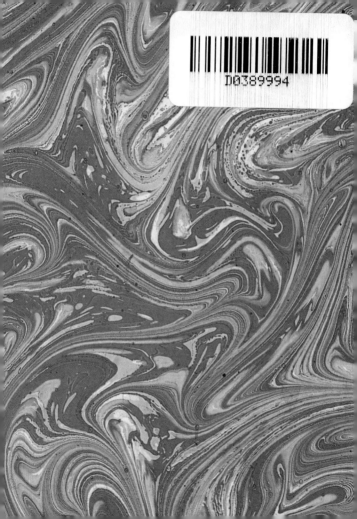

A *GARDEN* OF
HERBAL REMEDIES

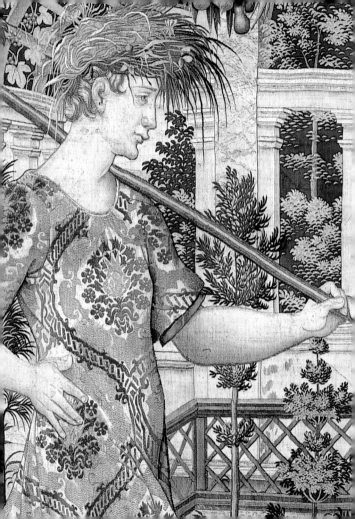

A GIFT OF HEALTH

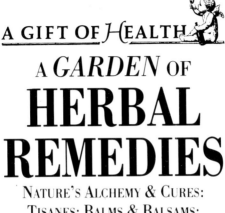

A *GARDEN* OF
HERBAL
REMEDIES

Nature's Alchemy & Cures:
Tisanes: Balms & Balsams:
Lotions & Potions, *Etc.*, *Etc.*

Compiled and
Visually Embellished
from Original Sources by
W. Craig Dodd Esq.

NH
NEW
HOLLAND

First published in the UK in 1996 by
New Holland (Publishers) Ltd
London • Cape Town • Sydney • Singapore

24 Nutford Place, London W1H 6DQ, UK

P.O. Box 1144, Cape Town 8000, South Africa

3/2 Aquatic Drive, Frenchs Forest, NSW 2086, Australia

ISBN 1 85368 670 0

Designed and edited by
Complete Editions
40 Castelnau, London SW13 9RU

Editor: Michèle Brown
Designer: Craig Dodd

Editorial Direction: Yvonne McFarlane
Reproduction by Hirt and Carter, Cape Town, South Africa
Printed and bound in Singapore by Tien Wah Press Pte Ltd

This is not a medical book. It is a gift book. It is not intended to
replace the services of a physician, nor is it meant to encourage
diagnosis and treatment of illness, disease or other medical
problems by the layman. Any application of the
recommendations set out in the following pages is at the reader's
discretion and sole risk. If under a physician's care, they will
advise if any recommendations are suitable for you. Pregnant
Women are advised to avoid all drugs – synthetic or herbal.

CONTENTS

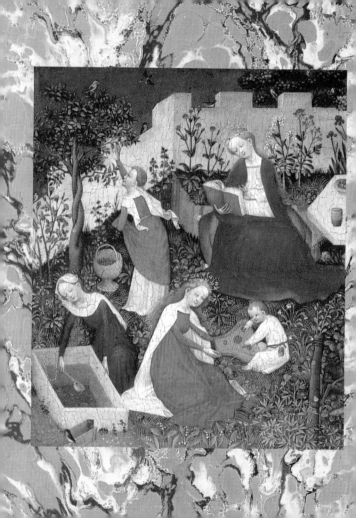

PREFACE

Within the pages of the Small Volumes which comprise of **A Gift of Health** there is contained the Collected Wisdom of Sages and Savants, Herbalists and Sensualists from throughout the Ages.

From their very Words the Modern Reader may glean much **Useful Information** to help with the **Problems of Everyday Life**, be they Physical or Psychological.

This very volume offers a Tantalising Insight into a Particular World of **Life Enhancing Wisdom** as do the Companion Volumes.

A Garden of Herbal Remedies takes you along the Pathways of the Healing Herbal Garden. The Wisdom of the Ancient Herbalists being distilled to illuminate this Healing Art. The Potency of Each and Every Herb herein is defined, together with a Veritable Pharmacopoeia of Nature's Remedies to lead to a Healthier Life.

A Compendium of Oriental Healing takes you into the Erudite World of the Ancient Healing Arts of the Orient. The Mysteries of Acupuncture, Meditation, Moxibustion and the Oldest of Herbal Cures are explained, together with the Ways of Ayurvedic Medicine which treats the Whole Person rather than an Isolated Disease.

A Bouquet of Aromatherapy is a Celebration of the Healing, Soothing and Sensual Qualities of the Plant Kingdom. It offers a Perfumed Voyage through the World of Essential Oils, their Uses, Practical applications and Healing Properties. It also features Dr. Bach's famed Flower Remedies and, on a lighter note, the Creation of Personal Pot-pourri and Fragrances.

A Cornucopia of Aphrodisiacs combines many Features of the aforesaid Companion Volumes, bringing together Folklore and Fancy, Enchanting Elixirs and Arousing Recipes to Enhance the Libido and Promote a Joyful Union of Partners.

Taken together, ingested and digested, the Messages from Across the Aeons of Time will truly prove to be **A Gift of Health**.

W. Craig Dodd

HERBS & HERBALISTS

herb *n.* **1.** plant of which the stem is not woody or persistent and which dies down to ground after flowering; plant of which leaves etc. are used for food, medicine, scent, flavour, etc. **2.** **~ bennet,** common avens (*Geum urbanum*) [prob. f. med. L *herba benedicta* blessed herb, as having expelled the Devil];

her'bal *a. & n.* (book with descriptions and account of properties) of herbs. [f. med. L *herbalis* (as prec.; see -AL)]

her'balist *n.* one skilled in herbs, esp. early botanical writer; dealer in medicinal herbs. [f. prec. + -IST]

Asked 'What is a herb?' the **Wise Emperor Charlemagne** replied 'The friend of the physician and the praise of cooks'

The Use of Plants to cure **Disorders** can be said to be older than the Human Race. Animals are naturally drawn to certain plants to cure illnesses and we can be sure that this practise goes back into the **Mists of Time**.

In tombs of the Neanderthal Age have been found **Pollen** and **Flowers** with the other **Remains**. These were thought to be Tributes, but it has been noted that they were all of Plants with Narcotic, and therefore, Healing Properties.

One of the earliest Herbalists was **John Gerard** who came from the County of Cheshire, England, and practised at the **Art of Chirugerie** in London. The most famous portrait of him shows him holding a spray of the Potato Plant and in the *Catalogue of Plants Growing in the London District of Holborn*, his home garden, he became the first to record the potato in print. His celebrated *Herball or Generall Histoire of Plants* was published in London in 1597. This is a Magnificently Coloured collection of hundreds of woodcut illustrations, each tinted by a Fair Hand.

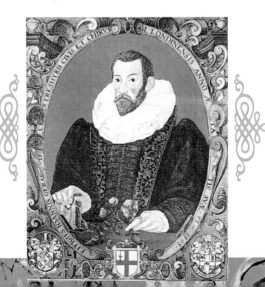

Such Ancient Herbals, and those which precede Gerard by many hundreds of years are the accumulated wisdom of near 2000 years by the Close Study of Plants. **Theophrastus** was *Enquiring into Plants* in the 3rd Century BC and advising that 'Basil be watered even at noon, for it is said that it grows more quickly if it be watered first with warm water'. **Dioscorides** of Anazarba wrote his *De Materia Medica* circa 60 AD and Pliny the Elder investigated *Naturall Histoire* (as translated in 1601) in 77 AD recording all manner of **Unusual Facts**. Macer's *Herbal* is a 12th century Middle English manuscript on which Anthony Askham based his *Lytel Herball* of 1550. The 15th century was particularly prolific for the production of Herbals. William Turner compiled his *New Herbal*, Thomas Hyll wrote *A Most Briefe and pleausant treatyse*, *The Proffitable Arte of Gardening* and *The Gardeners Labyrinth*, Thomas Tusser wrote *Five Hundred points of Good Husbandry* and Thomas Coghan *The Haven of Health*. Already Thomas Hyll was advising that 'chawinge of the fresh and grene parceleye' would sweeten the breath. The century ended with John Gerard's Great Work.

In the following century there is one Magisterial Work; *The English Physician Or an Astro-physical Discourse of the Vulgar Herbs of this Nation Being a Compleat Method of Physick whereby a man may preserve this Body in health; or cure himself being sick, for three pence charge, with such things one-ly as grow in England, they being most fit for English Bodies.* And so Culpeper's *Complete Herbal* was Conceived in 1652.

'Culpeper, the man that first ranged the woods and climbed the mountains in search of medicinal and salutary herbs, has undoubtedly merited the gratitude of posterity.'
Dr Johnson

In all this Time, the Herbs themselves remain Unchanged. Theophrastus, Pliny and Gerard described plants such as sage, mint and thyme which remain the same in form, height and colour as we know them Today.

'Hearbs are those whose root stalkles cannot be reckoned to be wood, but doe for the most part consist of Leaves, as *Fennel, Everlasting, Baulme, Mints & c.* The seed is that part of the Plant which is ended with a vitall faculty to bring forth its like, and it contains potentially the whole plant in it.

The Flower is the beauty of the Plant, arising from the most refined and concocted matter, and therefore is most commonly of a different colour . . .

The Leafe is that part of a Plant which is sent forth from the main stalks by another lesser stalk, and consists of three similar parts, to wit, veyns, sinnews and flesh . . .

The stalk is that part of a plant which riseth up from the root and is as it were a pipe to convey the nourishment . . .

The Root is the lowermost part of a plant, which, answers to the mouth in a man, and being fastened in the earth, drawes convenient nourishment unto it, and supplieth all its parts'

William Coles *The Art of Simpling* 1656

CONCOCTING & INFUSING

Herbal teas as **Medicinal Preparations** or indeed for **Simple Pleasure** can be made as **Infusions** or **Decoctions** depending upon the plant in question. For example, the Infusion Method should be employed when soft parts of the plant such as the Flowers, Leaves and non-woody Stems are used. Decoctions are used when Roots, Bark or Seeds are the Essential Ingredient.

INFUSIONS & TISANES

The simplest method of preparation consisting of little more than the addition of boiling water to the herb in question. The part of the plant being employed should be put in a **Warm Pot**, the boiling water poured over and then the pot should be covered. If you fail to do this essential oils will be lost in the steam which issues forth. Leave to infuse. There is no golden rule about the length of time. Personal Taste prevails, but beware excessive infusing as bitterness can result, no matter how sweet the herb. You will soon find out the most efficative strength for yourself. Children and Women with Child often prefer a Weaker Infusion, together with the addition of a more pleasing herb such as Mint or Balm to make it Palatable. If in doubt, consult a Herbal Practitioner.

For herbs which have a high Viscous or Mucilagineous content a Cold Water Infusion may be made. Comfrey is such a plant. This is a slow process as the chosen herb should be left to infuse in the cold water over-night.

One is well advised that Herbalists are of mixed minds over the ingestion of Comfrey. Some say we have no reason to fear its use, whilst others warn that it may incite serious disease.

DECOCTIONS

Woody parts of a plant require considerable heat to break them down into an **Administerable Potion**. They must be crushed or chopped into very small pieces and then added to a Fair Quantity of water in a Saucepan. Bring to the Boil and simmer for up to fifteen minutes.

TINCTURES

Tinctures are best produced professionally, but can be created in the home if so desired. The chosen herb is steeped in a mixture of **Water** and **Alcohol** to extract the **Healing Parts** of the herb and to preserve them.

In Suitable Proportions, deemed to be about five to one for standard tinctures, mix Water with the Alcohol of your choice, be it Vodka or Brandy. Add your herbs and seal in an airtight container and leave to Macerate for at least two weeks. Strain well through Muslin several times before use.

It is advisable to Take Advice when administering tinctures, especially to children. A suitable and highly palatable tincture for children can be made by replacing the Alcohol with Glycerol. Dilute with water or a fruit juice of your choice.

Tinctures make Effective Gargles and Mouthwashes and Throat Sprays when diluted with water before use.

HERBS FOR EXTERNAL USE & EFFECT

BATHS

Any of the aforementioned concotions, together with the Essential Oil of Suitable Herbs, can be added to your bath, whilst a muslin bag of fresh or dried aromatic herbs (in the Fashion of a Bouquet Garni) can be suspended below the hot water fawcet. The oil will be absorbed through the pores of the skin and the aromatic atmosphere will be inhaled.

Stronger admixtures of the above can give relief to aching feet and hands.

UNGUENTS & LOTIONS

These can be Laborious to make and are best acquired from **Herbal Practitioners**. If however you are so inclined they can be made at home. Here are two receipts of varying complexity.

Of the recommended herb or mixture of herbs take the prescribed amount. Finely chop and introduce into a vessel containing **Olive Oil** and **Beeswax** in the proportion of eight parts to one. Allow the mixture to soften through soaking and Heat Gently for a few moments in a *Bain Marie*, being explained as the vessel containing the mixture placed within another vessel containing warm water. The Effective Elements of the herb will be absorbed by the oil. Strain through muslin and pour into suitable Pots to allow to cool.

A simpler ointment can be made by adding a few drops of the prescribed Essential Oil to a Commercially Prepared pure vegetable face cream and mixing gently.

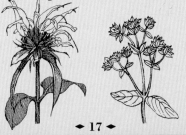

FOMENTATIONS

Poultices and Warm Compresses are widely used to relieve aches and pains. A **Poultice** is prepared by bruising and chopping the appropriate Herbs and Spices and mixing to a Paste with water. The mixture is placed in muslin and applied to the Afflicted Part. If convenient it should be kept warm with a Hot-Water Bottle. A **Warm Compress** is made by soaking a pad of Absorbent Material in the recommended mixture of Warm Infusions, Decoctions and Tinctures. The pad is then applied to the Afflicted Part. Cold Compresses can be fashioned in a similar mode, without warming the Ingredients.

There are many other Ways and Means of inhaling the Benificent Aromas of Herbs. Rooms can be easily deodorised by the addition of a few drops of an Essential Oil to a Plant spray, Atomiser, or sprinkled on Pot-Pourri. A further few drops can be added to a Herb Pillow to have by you to Induce Sleep.

ANCIENT LORE OF HERBS

The accumulated **Knowledge** of the **Use of Herbs** for **Medicinal Purposes** is a Combination of the Observation and the Wisdom of the Great Herbalists and Physicians. Some of their Concoctions, Decoctions, Lotions, Potions, Poultices and Pills have long been proved to be of a Fantastic and Fanciful Nature, but Modern Science has Sufficiently Proven the true worth of many of the Healing Plants. Their Usage of Old is described in the words of the Great Herbalists.

Agrimony is reputedly 'good for them with naughtie livers' according to Gerard the Herbalist, whose words hereafter are unascribed. The starry yellow flowers which cover the stems suggested to ancient herbalists its use in the healing of yellow jaundice. For Agrimony Tea pour boiling water over a mixture of Stems, Flowers and Leaves. Strain Well before using this Popular Tonic for Sore Throats and Weakness of the Bladder

Angelica has from Pagan Times been applied against Witchcraft and is efficaceous 'against the plague, and all corruptions taken by evil and corrupt aire.' Its magic powers are ascribed to Michael the Archangel whose feast day in the Pre-Gregorian Calendar fell on May 8 when Angelica was reputed to be in full bloom.

Anise, the seeds of which 'wasteth and consumeth winde, and is good against belchings' is recorded on the Tablets of Nineveh. In the 6th Century BC, Pythagoras held a spray in his hand to Prevent Epileptic Fits and Emperor Charlemagne included it in his Famed Herb Garden. Anise-flavoured liqueurs like Anisette and Turkish Raki warm the stomach and promote digestion.

Balm leaves, said Dioscorides, 'being drank with wine & also applied are good for the Scorpion smitten and ye dog-bitten'. It rivals Sage as a Prolonger of Life. Prince Llewellyn of Glamorgan lived to the Phenominal Old Age of 108 after following a diet of it. Balm tea made from an Infusion of the leaves is credited with help against fevers.

BEE STING

Bees cluster round Balm, thus increasing the chances of being stung when in close proximity to the plant. Just as dock grows near stinging nettles being a provedential antidote, so Balm's soothing leaves provide relief from stings. Extract the sting, taking Great Care not to squeeze yet more poison from it. Then rub the wound with Balm leaf.

Bay berries 'are very effectual against all poisons of venemous creatures, and the stings of wasps and bees' quoth Nicholas Culpeper. He also reports that 'Neither of witch nor devil nor lightning will hurt a man in a place where there stands a Bay Tree'. It is therefore Highly Advisable to have one standing near your doorway. It is alleged that chewing the leaves bestows the Gift of Prophecy, the Mild Narcotic effects of the Oil frequently producing Visions.

Its leaves were used to make garlands at the Pythian Games at Delphi; hence the title, Poet Laureate. The Bay Tree was sacred to Apollo in Greek Mythology for, when he was pursuing the Nymph Daphne, the Gods changed her into a Laurel Tree to escape him. From the leaves he wove a Garland.

Borage syrup 'comforethe the heart, purgeth Melancholie and quieteth the phrenticke or lunatickke person'. It is the herb of courage and gladness and Stimulates the Adrenal Juices. An infusion of the leaves Dried, or Fresh, soothes anguished throats.

THE POT OF BASIL

Basil 'taketh away sorrowfulness, which cometh of melancholie and make a man merrie and glad'. Its very name derives from the Greek *Basileus* meaning King hence, in France, it is known as the *Herbe Royale*. In Medieval Times a pot of Basil was placed in a window to show that the lady of the House was expecting a Lover. It is not recorded why a Lady should give such a Wanton Sign. In the Middle Ages Basil was strewn on the floor to keep away fleas and flies. To enhance the aroma, tear the leaves roughly, as cutting, in the Words of Richard Surflet, 'with any yron thinge', impairs the flavour.

In the *Decameron*, Boccaccio relates the Tragic Tale of Isabella, whose Young Lover is killed by her Brothers. She severed his head and kept it in a pot of basil by her bedside.

> She wrapped it up and for its tomb did choose
> A garden pot, wherein she laid it by
> And covered it with mould, and o'er it set
> Sweet Basil, which her tears kept ever wet.
>
> John Keats
> *Isabella, or, The Pot of Basil* 1818

Salome was thought to have preserved John the Baptist's Head in similar fashion.

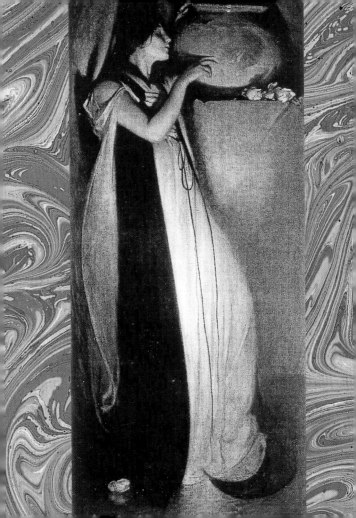

Burnet 'is a singular good herb for wounds; it staun-cheth bleeding inwardly taken or outwardly applied. In Wine it yeeldeth a certaiine grace in drinking'.

The King Kaba of Hungary knew of these Powers and Properties and during a battle with his brother used Burnet juice to staunch the wounds of fifteen thousand of his Soldiers. Chewing the leaves freshens the breath.

Caraway seeds confected 'with Sugar into Confits, are very good for the stomacke, help digestion and asswage and dissolve all windiness'. Traditionally Carraway was eaten with apples.

Nay, you shall see my orchard, where in an arbour, we will eat a last year's pippin of my own graffing, with a dish of carraways . . .'
Shallow to Falstaff Henry IV
Wm Shakespeare Esq

Superstition has it that apart from medicinal properties Caraway has Magical Properties. Objects containing it could not be taken away or stolen. And thus pigeons were fed Caraway to Ensure their return. Likewise a few seeds placed by a wife into her husband's pocket would stop him being lured away.

Chamomile appears in many Herbals and the 'Most Friendly and Beneficial Herb' having Many Applications. Because of its persistent growing qualities it is associated with Youth.

   ...For though the chamomile, the more it is trodden on, the faster it grows, yet youth, the more it is wasted the sooner it wears'
   Falstaff to King Hal, *Henry IV Part 1*
   Wm Shakespeare Esq

It is Efficaceous for Digestive Upsets, Colicky Pains and, Applied Externally, soothes Sores and Burns. An Inhalation eases Asthma and Hay Fever. ·

Comfrey root 'made in a posset of ale, and given to drink againste the paine in the back, gotten by any violent motion, as wrestling, or overmuch use of women' will achieve a perfect cure in but four or five days.

   Known over the Centuries as Knitbone and Bruise-wort for its capacity to Heal Wounds and Internal Ulcers, External Use for Grazes, Cuts and Bruises is Highly Recommended, but for Internal Ailments Judicious Use and Caution are Advised. Comfrey Baths In Folklore, were popular on Wedding Night to restore virginity. It is of Particular Importance to those who will eat nothing originating from the Animal Kingdom.

CAT'S DELIGHT

Catnip, or Catmint has By Repute been attractive to cats since the Fourteenth Century when Agnus Castus wrote 'The vertu of this herbe is if a cat ete thereof it shall bryne forthe kytlyngss anon'. In the Seventeenth Century William Coles recorded in his *Art of Simpling* 'When the Cat is sick he goes to the Nep or Catmint'.

Cats become Even More Playful with a Catnip Mouse. From Butter Muslin cut out two Mouse Shapes. Partly sew the edges, fill with Dried Catnip and complete sewing.

The Sweat Inducing qualities of Catnip make it effectual for Chills and Influenzas. It relieves Congestion of the Nasal Passages and is Valuable for Colicky Pains. Its Leafy Tops make a Digestive Tea.

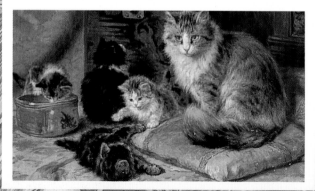

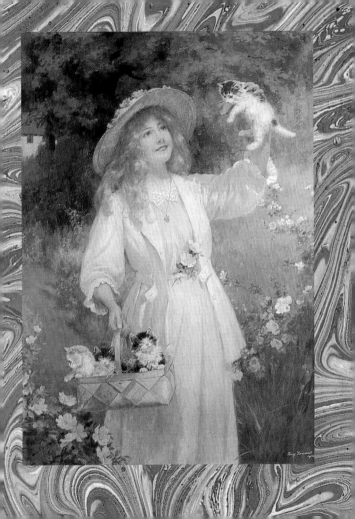

Dandelion 'helpeth to procure rest and sleep to bodies distempered by the heat of ague-fits, and the distilled water of it is effectual to drink in Pestilential Fevers' according to Nicholas Culpeper, who also records that it is 'Vulgarly called piss-a-beds'.

Praised for providing a Pair of Medicinal Effects; the Leaf increases passage of water whilst the Root gently eases the Stool and is a Tonic for the Liver.

Dill is recorded as 'a gallant expeller of wind' in *The English Physician* of 1652 it also 'stayeth the hiccough being boyled in wine and but smelled unto,'

Unusual in the Community of Herbs, it takes its name from the Norse, *dilla* meaning 'to lull' and is still a Homely Remedy to soothe babies suffering from the aforesaid Wind.

Hyssop, in the time of Culpeper was 'so universally known that I consider it needless to give of any description'. In these times it is Noted Principally as an ingredient of Chartreuse. It is also cultivated to encourage bees, giving their Honey a particular Aroma and Potency. The medicinal qualities of Honey are universally recognised. Hyssop Tea has long been a Country Cure for colds, phlegm and rheumatism.

Lavender 'is refreshing to them that have the Catalepsie and them that have the falling sickness and that use to swoune'. Culpeper adds that 'Lavender is little used in inward physicke, but outwardly, the oyle for cold and benumbed parts, and the dryed flowers to comfort and dry up the moisture of a cold braine'

Its medicinal use was recorded by Dioscorides as good for Troubles of the Thorax and from the sixteenth century it has been used as a cure for sore throats. Externally Oil of Lavender can ease aches and pains and for swabbing wounds. It is also an excellent aid for the Soothing of Burns whilst at the same time reducing the chances of Unsightly Scars.

Lavender Tea is Good for Headaches and Overcoming Faintness, causing Sweating which in turn rids the body of poisonous toxins through the pores.

For Common Folk it has always been a Mainstay to Scent Country Gardens.

Fennel seed in Powder Form 'drunke for certaine daies together fasting preserveth the eyesight; whereof was written;

> Of Fennell, Roses, Vervaine, Rue and Celandine
> Is made a water good to clear the seight of eine

According to Sophocles, Prometheus stole the Spark of Fire from Olympus and brought it back to earth in a Giant Stalk of Fennel. It was used to give Strength, Courage and Long Life.

Charlemagne planted it in his Herb Garden and it was used on Fast Days to Dull the Appetite. Hence its Inclusion in Reducing Diets.

> Above the lowly plants it towers,
> The fennel with its yellow flowers,
> And in an earlier age than ours,
> Was gifted with the wondrous powers,
> Lost vision to restore,
> It gave new strength and fearless mood
> And gladiators, fierce and rude,
> Mingled it in their daily food,
> And he who battled and subdued,
> A wreath of fennel wore
>
> *The Goblet of Life* Henry W. Longfellow

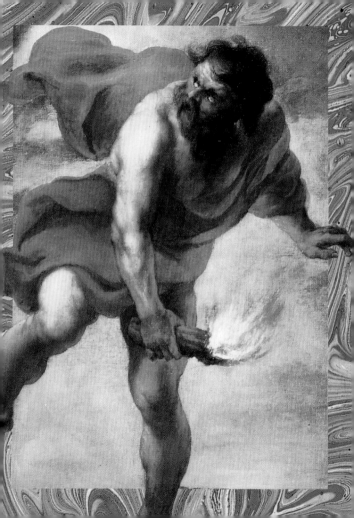

Marigold petals 'are dried and kept throughout Dutch-land against winter, to put into brothes, in Physicall potions and for divers other purposes'. In these Times they include skin ailments such as Wounds, Grazes and Minor Burns. A Tincture on an Eyepad eases Conjunctivitis, and taken as a Gargle it Heals Mouth Ulcers. The Astringent Quality staunches bleeding and promotes healing cuts, bruises, cold sores and warts. In the Great War soldiers kept Marigold Leaves in their pack for just such a purpose.

> The distilled water of Marigolds put into the eyes
> cureth the rednesse and inflammation of the same
> *A Niewe Herball* 1578

Marjoram was 'a remedie against cold diseases of the braine and head, being taken any way; put up the nosthrils it provoketh sneesing, and draweth foorth much baggage flegfme; it easeth the toothach being chawed' The Essential Oil of Marjoram is still used to Alleviate Toothache. It is also used to soothe Sprains and Bruises. Sweet Majoram was a symbol of happiness put on graves for a cheerful farewell to the Near and Dear. Marjoram Tea is good for headaches.

Meadowsweet 'doth calm the minde' It has many of the Uses of Newfangled Medicinal Aids such as Aspirin, but without the Concomitant evil side effects.

Mint 'smell', saith, Pliny 'doth stir up the mind, and the taste to a greedy desire of meat. Mint is marvellous wholesome for the stomacke. It is good against watering eies'. It is named after the Nymph Minthe who was beloved by Pluto. He had not regarded the Jealousy of Persephone, Queen of Hades, who turned her into sweetsmelling mint doomed to wait until Eternity at the entrance to the Dark Underwold ruled by Pluto. For centuries it has been used in baths and funerals alongside Rosemary and Myrtle to hide the Odour of Decay. In the fourteenth century it was used for whitening teeth and to this day is employed in the Manufacture of Toothpastes and Mouthwashes. Peppermint has the remarkable qualities of being both hot and cold. When ingested it induces heat, being a good tonic during Convalescence after Debilitating Illness. It is cool when applied externally.

They lay it with good success unto the styngings of Bees and Wasps. *A Niewe Herball* 1578

Nasturtium, the 'Nose-Twister' with its hot peppery taste and small is named from the Latin *Nasus* 'nose' and *tortus* 'twisted' by Pliny He also noted that a sluggish man should eat it to arouse him from the state of torpor. Taken in Salads it is a Prime Source of Vitamin C.

Oregano 'or Bastard Marjoram . . . given in wine is remedie against the bitings and stingings of venemous beastes and cureth them that have drunk Opium or the juice of the blacke Poppie or Hemlocke'. More common uses are for the treatment of 'scabs, itchings and scurvinesse'. It also, according to Culpeper, 'helps the cough and lungs, cleanseth the Body of Choller expelleth poyson and remedieth the infirmities of the spleen'. Taken as an infusion it is good to settle the stomach.

Pennyroyal 'worne around the head is of great force against the swimming of the head, the paines and giddines thereof'. Named after the Latin word for 'flea' it is noted for repelling them. The same applies for lice, flies, mosquitoes, moths and ants. Macerate the leaves and rub onto exposed skin to test this effect.

The potentially poisonous qualities of pennyroyal oil make it most imperative that you avoid ingesting the oil or using it in an overly concentrated dose as an infusion. Women with Child are advised to avoid all contact with pennyroyal.

FOR GOOD OR EVIL

Parsley 'taketh away the stinking of the breath, especially from such as have drunke much wine or eaten garlike'. So wrote Richard Surfleet in the *Countrie Farme* of 1600. It is also one of the most Potent medicinal herbs, a handful containing a greater profusion of Vitamin C than a single orange. This makes it ideal for those with a Deficiency of Iron or suffer from Weak Blood. It relieves Rentention of Fluid and helps Elimate Noxious Poisons from the Body, a Great Relief for those suffering Gout and Arthritis. A Decoction of Parsley Seeds may prove effective in Lightening the Load of the Headache, Migraine and Asthma. Juice of Parsley alleviates Toothache.

Dedicated to Persephone, Queen of Hades there is a Dark Aspect in the History of Parsley. Greek funeral wreaths were made of it and it was considered Unlucky to transplant it from one house to another. To do so would Induce Abortion to the Woman of the House. To this day Parsley is not advised during Pregnancy.

As Parsley is slow to germinate, folklore records that it 'goes seven times to the Devil and back'. Perhaps it was for this reason that it became an important ingredient of the unguent concocted by witches to enable them to fly.

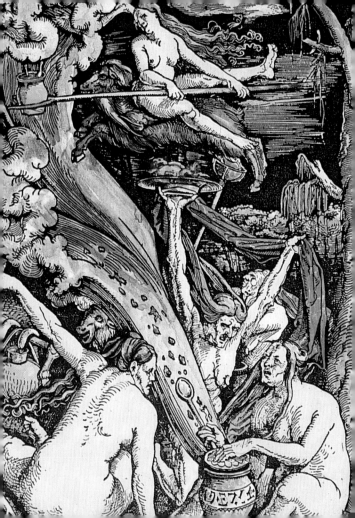

Rue 'eaten with the kernels of Walnuts or figs stamped together and made into a masse or paste is good against evill aires, the pestilence or plague'. It has long since had a reputation as an Antidote to Poison. It is said to be the herb which protected Ulysses from the magic used by Circe to turn his men into swine. The first Duke of Saxony used rue as a mark of heraldry which today has devolved into the Suit of Clubs in Playing Cards.

♣ ♣ ♣ ♣ ♣ ♣ ♣ ♣ ♣ ♣ ♣

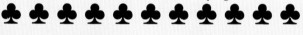

Sage 'is singular good for the head and braine; it quickenth the sences and memory . . . takes away shaking of the members; and being put into the nostrils, it draweth fine flegme from the head'. Once used as a substitute for Tobacco. Sage Infusion, used as a gargle when cool is used to Whiten the Teeth and Strengthen the Gums. Sage tooth-powder, made by grinding sage leaves and sea salt together, removes yellow stains from the teeth.

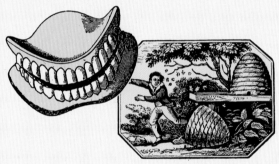

Savory 'saith Dioscorides, maketh thinne, and doth marvellously prevail against winde: therefore it is with good success boiled and eaten with beanes, peason, and other windie pulses'. Rubbed on bee-stings it gives hasty relief from pain.

OPHELIA'S GARLAND

Rosemary 'floures being drunke at morning and evening
first and last, taketh away the stench of the mouth and
breath, and make it very sweet.'

> Rosemary is for remembrance
> Between us daie and night;
> Wishing that I might alwaies have
> You present in my sight.
> *A Nosegaie* 1584

Rosemary is for remembrance and for memory as, taken
in Infusion, it Increases the flow of Blood to the head
Stimulating the Brain. It also dispels Winter Colds,
improves Circulation and helps Digestive Disorders.

> There's rosemary, that's for remembrance;
> pray, love, remember:
> and there is Pansies, that's for thought's . . .
> There's Fennel for you, and Columbines:
> – we may call it herb-grace o'Sundays
> . . . O, you must wear your rue with a difference.
> – There's a daisy:
> . . . I would give you some violets, but they
> withered all when my father died . . .
> *Hamlet*
> Wm. Shakespeare Esq

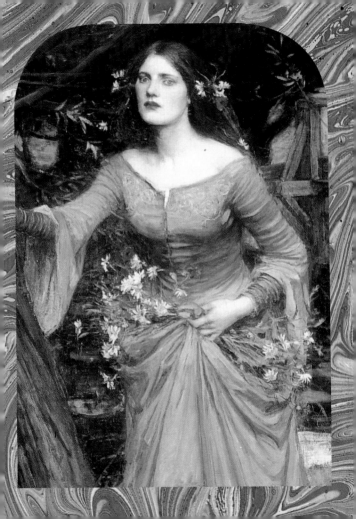

Strawberry leaves 'boyled & applied in manner of a pultis taketh away the burning heate in wounds: the decoction thereof strengthneth the gums, fastneth the teeth and is good to be helde in the mouth, both against the inflammation or burning heate thereof'. In olden days the leaves were added to cooling drinks. And as an Infused Cooling Astringent used for fevers. Teeth were cleaned with strawberry juice. Symbolically the fruit of righteousness as depicted in Botticelli's Venus and Virgin Mary.

Tansy 'is good for the stomacke. For if any bad humours cleave therunto, it doth perfectly concoct them and scowre them downwards.' Culpeper used it 'to cleanse and heal ulcers in the mouth or secret parts . . . and wonderfully cools the hot fits of agues'. Tansy should be approached with **Caution** as it is not only Bitter to the Modern Taste, but is also an Irritant Narcotic and should be used Sparingly. Tansy tea, infused from but Part of a Leaf may be Taken Sparingly for Gout.

Tarragon, Culpeper reminds his readers, 'that no serpent will meddle with him that carried this Herb,' which makes it invaluable to those sojourning in Rural Areas. It was used to ease toothaches by the Romans and throughout Araby. It calms those of a Nervous Disposition particularly when that Condition encourages Slow Digestion.

Thyme 'when boyled in water and hony and drunken is good against a hard and painful cough and shortness of breath', according to the *Niewe Herbal* of 1578. There are in Excess of Sixty Varieties of this herb and they make a veritable Herb Garden in themselves. It is an ingredient of many Cough Linctuses, Creams. Lotions, Potions, and Mouthwashes. It has at various times been used to Combat the dreaded Typhoid and Anthrax in Ruminants.

During the Wars of the Roses Lancastrian Ladies embroided a bee hovering over a sprig of thyme to present as a Memento to their Menfolk when setting out to battle.

Violets 'are good for all inflammations, especially of the sides and lungs; they take away the hoarseness of the chest, the ruggedness of the winde-pipe and jawes'. Use in pottages and conserves to provide Vitamin C and as an infusion are Beneficial to the Kidneys.

Wormwood 'is very profitable to those troubled with choler, for it cleanseth thorough his bitterness, purgeth by siege: by reason of the binding qualities, it strengtheneth and comforteth.' This bitter herb was used in the making of the Liqueur favoured by the French, Absinthe, which when taken Habitually causes paralysis and death. It should be used only under the most careful instruction as over-use can cause Hallucinations.

Yarrow 'is a principal herb for all kinde of bleedings, and to heal up new and old ulcers and greene wounds.' It is named after the Golden-haired Achilles who employed it to Staunch a spear Wound sustained by his Comrade, Telephus, during the Trojan Wars. It is also, By Repute, claimed to similarly staunch Nosebleeds. Like Marigold petals it was carried as a medicinal aid by Soldiers in the Great War. Taken internally it stimulates the Appetite. Its healing properties soothe Gastric and Enteric Infections. Chewing the leaves of Yarrow is Nature's Way of alleviating extreme toothache.

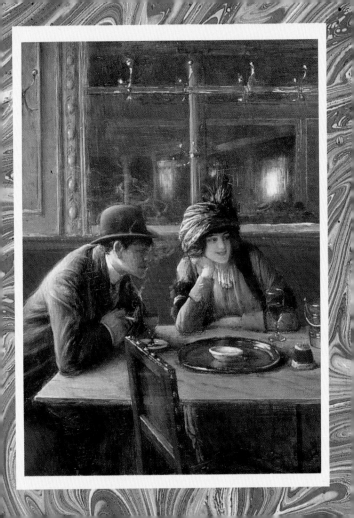

A Little Sip Of Herb Tea

Herbal Teas have long been known for their Therapeutic and Medicinal qualities – at times Stimulating, Soothing, Invigorating and for Relaxation. By Precise Definition all teas are Herb Teas as the China or Indian Tea with which we are familiar are Simple Infusions of the leaves of *Camellia sinensis*

Herb Leaves used in teas may be Fresh or Dried, though it is advisable to use Half the Quantity of the dried herb. Fresh leaves produce an extra aroma. The Advised Proportion is to use two to three teaspoons of fresh herb leaves to a Sufficiency of Boiling Water to provide an infusion to your taste.

The Preferred Method is to place the Chosen Herb in a warm teapot. Freshly boiled water is poured on top. If the water is Vilely Cholorinated use a Natural Still Mineral Water to obtain the True Taste of the Herb. Allow the tea to brew for three to five minutes, then pour the Liquor through a strainer into the Cup or Glass. But beware! If a glass is your choice a spoon must first be placed in it to avoid unfortunate Cracking. A Slice of Lemon may be your Wish and if a sweetener is required, stir in a Modicum of Clear Honey.

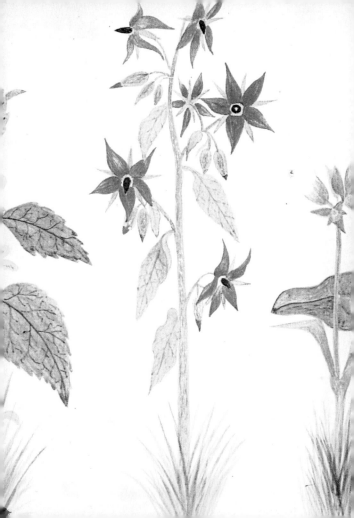

For the Purest of Flavours it is essential that the teapot should be Scrupulously Clean. A Glass Teapot is recommended, providing an infusion to please both the Palate and the Eye.

When Adventuring on the Road to Consumption of Herb Teas acquaint your palate with teas made from a single herb before Embarking on the Blending of Herbs.

AN ALPHABET OF HERBS FOR TEA

Angelica – Use the leaves alone or with a tiny strip of lemon zest. It is pale green and rather Bitter, like China tea. Efficaceous for the Relief of Colds.

Basil – Use the leaves alone or add two to a pot of Assam tea. Basil and Sage tea is also Most Flavoursome.

Bergamot – Fresh or dried flower heads make a Useful addition to a pot of green China Tea

Betony – A Delicious Infusion may be made from the leaves. The addition of a short strip of Orange or Lemon zest, a piece of Cinnamon Bark or a few cloves is Highly Recommended. Culpeper claims it an excellent remedy for sick hogs.

Chamomile – A Very Common herb which is an Aid to Slumber for the Relief of Rheumatism and, when cooled, as a Face Wash for a clear complexion.

Caraway – A Mild-tasting tea can be infused from fresh leaves and can Prove Efficaceous for Improving the Digestion.

Elderflower – A Particularly Fragrant tea may be made from fresh or dried flowers. Culpeper claimed it can help '. . . the gout, piles, inflammations of the eyes and the biting of serpents or mad dogs . . .'

Fennel – The leaves, flowers and seed can be used to make teas of Varying Strengths. John Gerard wrote that 'The pouder of the seed of Fennell drunke for certaine daies together fasting preservth the eyesight'

Fenugreek – Dried seeds are used, but they must be bruised in a Mortar before infusing.

Hawthorn – Freshly plucked leaves give the True Taste of the Hedgerow.

Hibiscus – Use fresh and dried flowers Enhanced by the addition of a bruised Cardomon pod.

Hyssop – Best made with fresh leaves and a strip of orange zest. Use only a few leaves as it is Spicy and Resinous. It is effacaceous for Colds, Phelgm and Mucus. When cold it can also be used to bathe Bruises and Black Eyes.

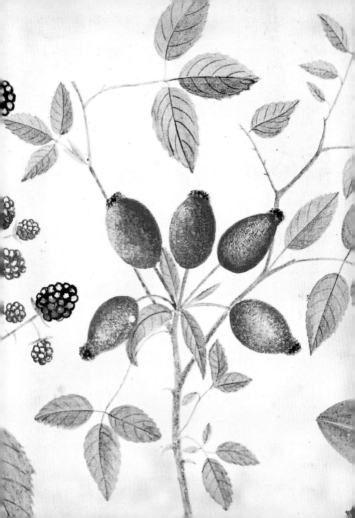

Lemon Balm – Use fresh leaves and sweeten with Honey. It is Credited with clearing the Head and Alleviating Fevers. Infused with Marjoram it was traditionally served to Cows for Strength after Calving.

Lemon Verbena – Soothing Properties when added to a Pot of China Tea.

Lime-Flower – Clean, Refreshing and Invigorating.

Mint – All Varieties make an Excellent Infusion. Used for Medicinal Purposes since Antiquity, for its Refreshing Taste and Calming Effect on the Stomach.

Rose – Fresh or Dried Hips or Petals make a most Pleasing Beverage. Rose-hip tea has a remarkably high Concentration of Vitamin C.

Rosemary – An Aromatic Tea, taken with Lemon Juice and Honey to Your Taste. It is said to Alleviate Headaches.

Sage – An Infusion of Sage can be good for the Liver and Against Fevers. Cooled, it can be used as a Gargle to Whiten Teeth and Strengthen Gums

Thyme – Each Variety of Thyme has a Distinctive Aroma from Pepper to Pineapple. Good for Easing Sore Throats

A Veritable Pharmacopoeia
Of Herbal Remedies

A host of Everyday Ailments from an **Excessive Acidity of the Stomach** to **Unsightly Warts** can be alleviated by the judicious use of **Herbal Compounds**. The Remedies described herein are a General Guide which Sufferers can prepare themselves. **Specific Doses** should be sought from **Herbal Practitioners** or Reputable **Homeopathic Suppliers**.

Acidity of the Stomach

It is advised that a cup of Chamomile tea, infused with a few fresh Mint leaves or indeed a pinch of dried Mint, will alleviate this unpleasantness. Should the symptoms recur with Renewed Ferocity, medical advice should be obtained.

Tightening of the Chest

Chest pain can occur when there is a shortage of oxygen in the muscles of the heart. A Brief Attack after a period of exercise, a reaction to Strong Emotions or living at High Altitudes, can be relieved with an infusion of Sage and Lime flowers in a glass of water. Persistent or Spreading pains should be carefully investigated.

Halitosis

Pungent breath can be sweetened, but not cured, with Common Herbal Remedies such as chewing Parsley or drinking Peppermint Tea.

Bruising of the Skin

Light bruising of the skin after a Fall or a Blow which does not result in an open wound can be bathed in distilled Witch Hazel. This not only heals, but acts as an effective Skin Cleanser.

Corns

This troublesome and oft-times painful hard, dead tissue within the outer layer of the skin is mostly alleviated by the attentions of a Chiropodist. In recent years it has been discovered during Medical Trials that material from Marigold plants, manufactured by Homeopathic Practitioners, can be effective after only one application.

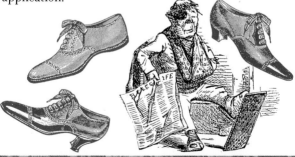

FOLLICULAR DEPRIVATION

For those Concerned about **Alopecia**, the Loss of Hair, the Herbal Medicine Chest can provide much hope. The Herbal Kitchen too can play it's part as the State of the Inner man and Woman plays an important part in Invigorating the Hair.

Eggs can provide nourishment both Internally and Externally. A nourishing foodstuff ingested in many ways, eggs can provide a wholesome Lotion for the hair. Take one egg and mix with a little water. Apply to the hair, cover and leave overnight.

An equally efficaceous and equally glutinous lotion can be prepared from two handfuls each of Watercress and Nettles. Pound in a pestle and Mortar to a thick paste and apply to the hair. This should be left on the hair for two hours before washing out.

The most efficaceous herb to take internally is Parsley, which improves the blood suppy to the cranium. Used externally, the freshly squeezed juice adds lustre to hair. Rosemary, too, also improves the circulation.

Lavender and Rosemary Infused in hot water for three hours, cooled and applied to the hair has been tested over the years. The addition of Sage can make it even more useful.

Used singly, infusions of Chamomile, Burdock and Yarrow have been noted by Great Herbalists for preserving the natural beauty of the hair, its length and thickness etc etc. Ultimately, with Sincere Regret, it has to be recorded that even Nature at her Most Persuasive cannot stop hair loss if it has been your misfortune to Inherit this Unhappy Condition.

Dandruff is an Unslightly and Irritable Condition in which dead skin cells are shed from the scalp in greater amounts than is normal. It is often associated with Oily Skin or a great Intake of Sugar, thus depleting the quantities of Vitamin B the body requires. Whilst an increased intake of Vitamin B and the application of Vitamin E oil ease the Condition, Herbs can play Nature's Part in a Cure; a Daily Application of an infusion of Rosemary and Sage in water being most effective.

Dry Eyes Soreness and Dryness of the Eyes and a Temporary Inability to produce Tears can be a great irritation. The widely available Evening Primrose Oil, taken As Instructed, can be a great relief.

Waxing of the Ears

If there is Pain in the Ears or Impaired Hearing the cause may prove to be an Accumulation of Wax. The commonest aid is warm Olive Oil inserted prior to syringing. However an Alternative is the use of Warm Almond Oil nightly for about seven days. This will perform the same function as olive oil and may well remove some of the offending wax altogether.

Strain of the Eyes

Tiredness of the Eyes through excessive reading, unsuitable lighting or close attention to the new-fangled invention, the Visual Display Unit, results in much discomforture. An eyebath of five chamomile heads in an ample quantity of water will provide much relief.

Heartburn

Over-indulgence at the Groaning-Board may result in Unpleasant Sensations in the Oesophagus. Less serious attacks can be alleviated by two cups of an infusion of five to eight pinches of Aniseed to a fair quantity of water.

Hiccoughs

If after Sipping a glass of Water the exhausting symptoms persist, a cup of Sage Tea, comprising one teaspoon of Sage to a cup of water, should be sipped slowly. This Remedy was not brought to the attention to Pope Pius XII who died from an Excessive Attack of Hiccoughs.

THE RAVAGES OF ALCOHOL

Let us have wine and women, mirth and laughter …
Sermons and Soda Water the day after.
Lord Byron

Plain Water is most efficaceous in Reducing the after-effects of Imbibing Great Quantities of Alcohol. A large quantity should be drunk before retiring after a Night of Excess.

Should symptoms persist there is a variety of Herbal and Vegetable Remedies available. Intense Headaches and Nausea can be Relieved with Vitamin B Complex together with Evening Primrose Capsules and a Glass of Water. To avoid such Unpleasantness it may prove effective to take a similar concoction at least one hour before embarking on further Alcoholic Excesses.

Ancient Greeks believed such troubles were caused by noxious fumes rising to the head. Consequently they wore wreathes of violets, myrtle and roses on their heads and decorated the wine jars with such flowers.

The Decoction of Violets is good against hiate fevers and inflammations of the liver
A Niewe Herball

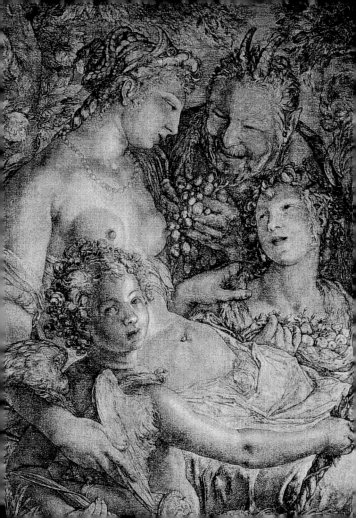

A sluggish Liver is calmed by an Infusion of Rosemary and Irritations of the Stomach calmed by Mint, Chamomile or Rosehip Teas. Cabbage Juice or Salad is also effective. Prune or grapefruit juice clean the liver. Galen the Greek recommended fomentations of Cabbage Juice and to wrap the brow in cabbage leaves. Aristotle suggested the same.

> Last evening you were drinking deep,
> So now your head aches. Go to sleep;
> Take some cabbage boiled when you wake
> And there's an end of your headache
> Athenaeus of Naucratis

If you are Afflicted by the Gout after Intemperance with Good Port Wine a decoction of Comfrey gives some relief. A similar Decoction of Eucalyptus, brought from Australasia in the middle of the nineteenth century, is equally efficative. Cherries clear the Kidneys and Watercress aids the body to expel unpleasant acids. Queen Elizabeth of Hungary cured herself of Gout at the great age of 72, so effectively restoring her beauty that the King of Poland offered his hand in marriage. The Receipt is to be found on a later page.

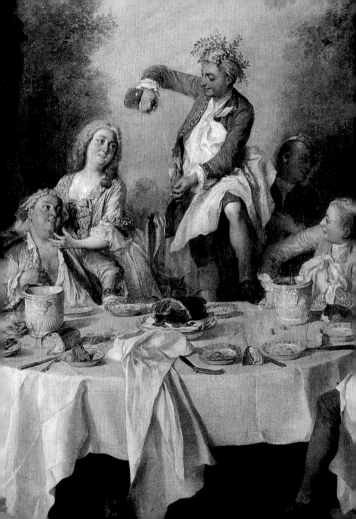

NO MOVEMENT & AN ILL WIND

'The decoction of Dill, be it herbs or seeds, in white wine, being drunke, it is a gallant expeller of winde'
Nicholas Culpeper

Herbs provide a whole battery of Remedies for two most inconvenient conditions, the one Uncomfortable and the other the Cause of Much Embarrassment if in Polite Company. As society has changed the Noble Fart is not acceptable as 'twas when the Great Herbalists gave many Concoctions to encourage such Bodily Functions. In these Modern Times Preparations to Restrain are more in Favour.

No Matter that, but the difficult passage of Stool has always been and remains a painful Affliction. It is Unfortunate that many of the remedies for this Latter Condition providing welcome relief exacerbate the former condition. A Tincture of Fennel is a Great Aid to Evacuation, but it also Encourages Flatulence.

Mild Constipation has many and varied cures. Cinnamon tea after cold food, as with ginger, parsley, relaxes. Pulses and Beans provide much needed fibre, but alas there is an excess of Flatulence. Sweet Almond Oil is Pleasant Medicament without the Unfortunate Effects Previous.

For Chronic Constipation the coating of Plantain seeds form a jelly-like substance to ease evacuation; they were also effective against mad dogs. Globe Artichoke also Lubricates the Great Intestine. Chamomile, which was used to cure the ague in Egyptian times regulates peristalsis thus being effective to cure the two extreme Conditions of Constipation and excess bowel movement. For greatly excessive movements Marigolds have long been a recognised cure as has a decoction of Hawthorn Bark. Eucalyptus, the Fever Tree, is also efficaceous.

An Infusion of Lavender calms the digestive tract with a concomitant reduction of Flatulence, whilst Apples harmonise the system, so helping both conditions.

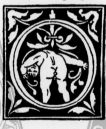

Insomnia

Debilitating Lack of Sleep caused by Anxiety can be most successfully treated with a host of Homeopathic Products which are readily available. For those who wish to make their own infusion a pinch each of Lime flowers, Vervain (Verbena) and Marjoram in a glass of hot water will induce Drowsiness.

Travel Sickness

The Undulation of Waves or the Motion of your Carriage can cause a Disturbance of the Balance Organ of the Inner Ear resulting in Nausea and Vomiting. The Most Effective Herbal Cure is to acquire Capsules of powdered Ginger to take before Commencing your Journey.

Nosebleed

A sudden onset of Epistaxis, for that is the correct term, can cause Great Embarrassment. They can be Staunched by the application of Gauze, but for Greater Effectiveness this should be moistened with an infusion of Yarrow, which every Judicious Traveller carries.

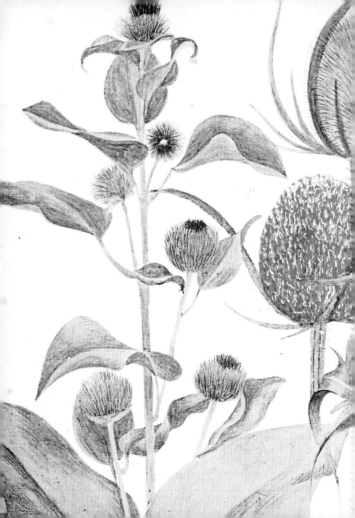

ARDOUR IMPAIRED

'Ginger being ruled by Venus transforms
Frigid Women into temptresses'
Nicholas Culpeper

Effective Herbs and Spices have long been Sought to Improve Sexual Potency. The Ancient Herbalists believed that they had Knowledge of Miraculous Cures and related Tales of Astounding Reinvigouration.

We must now be More Circumspect in our View of these Matters. Cinnamon was valued higher than gold in the Ancient World, such was the Belief in its power as an Aphrodisiac and Renewer of Sexual Energy. A Porridge of Exotic Cinnamon with Simple Oats is regarded as being something of a 'tonic for the female parts' and impaired Sterility and Impotence.

Ginger, so Highly Spoken of by Culpeper, reinvigorates the reproductive system by making up a deficiency of body warmth. Rose, the Symbol of Love, is widely used in the treatment of Female Diseases. The Petals act as a Decongestant of the Female Reproductive System and Enhance Fertility and Sexual Desire. They are an important Weapon in the Armoury to Fight Impotence in Men. They can be ingested as Teas, Tinctures or Jellies.

Impotency may not have a Physiological Cause, but may result from Anxiety or Emotional and Physical Tension. Herbal Remedies are Legion to Relieve Tension and advice should be taken.

From the Kitchen Garden healthy Juices may be prepared. An effective mixture is said to be the juice of Red Cabbage, Celery and Lettuce in Proportions to your taste.

The Homeopathic Remedy is *Agnus Castis* if the onset of an Impotent Condition is noticed, with *Lycopdium* for a more Serious Condition. If it is thought the Condition is the result of Anxiety *Argent. nit.* is recommended.

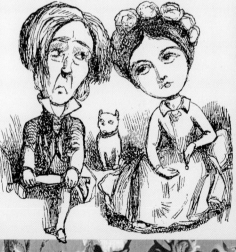

Rash

Mild Rashes unassociated with Specific Complaints may be soothed by the application of pure Aloe Vera Jelly after bathing the Affected Parts.

Inflammation of the Eye

Plebeian types call this condition Pink-Eye, as the whites of the eye redden through the Activities of Bacteria. A Marigold or Cornflower eyebath may prove Most Effective.

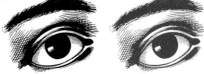

Stye of the Eye

This Unsightly and Irritating Boil on the Follicle of an Eyelash can be treated with an eyebath made from Chamomile Heads and ample water.

Warts

Many ritual Charms exist to remove these Benign Tumours under the outer skin layer. When successful they prove the power of Mind over Body. Herbal Remedies include the Application of a slice of Garlic or Celandine juice to the affected Area.

PASSAGE OF THE MOON

The Moon Goddess is the protector of childbirth, regulator of tides and the flow of life. The Female Cycle is the same length as the Period between Two Full Moons.

At the Onset of the Cycle there can be Great Stress. An Infusion of Various herbs can help, but care with Diet is also recommended. Foods which Irritate the Liver should be avoided, as should Hot Spices, Alcohol and Coffee. Highly refined Sugar should be replaced by one of Nature's Sweeteners. Refined Grains should also be taken in modest quantity.

Herbal remedies include Lemon Balm which can relieve Mental Stress and Physical Cramps. Rose used as Infusion or Essential Oil calms the Liver and Strengthens the Pancreas especially from Mid-Cycle to the End of the Cycle.

Evening primrose oil can give Great Relief if taken ten days before the Period in Conjunction with varying quantities of herbal mixtures taken from Chamomile, Lemon Balm and Marigold.

If the Cycle is not completed it is Essential to Assess that this is not through any natural Cause to be determined by your Physician. A tea or tincture of

Mugwort or Sage may be taken once a week for three weeks to bring on the Cycle. A Sage and Rosemary massage may induce Regularity of the Cycle. Such treatments should be applied for no more than three months. Excessive Flow on Completion of the Cycle is affected by hyperactivity of the liver and gall bladder according to Chinese Lore. Similar infusions, as already referred to, are effective as are Infusions or Tinctures of Lady's Mantle or Marigold.

Comfrey 'is good to be applied to Womens Breasts that grow sore by the abundance of Milk . . .'

Nicholas Culpeper

THE CHANGE OF LIFE

The many and varied Uncomfortable Conditions which accompany this important phase of a Woman's Life can be Alleviated by Herbal and Floral Preparations. Hot Flushes, Excessive Perspiration, Palpitations and Dryness are often the cause of an Overheated Liver. Taken as Teas or Tinctures, Roses, Violets, Sage, alone or mixed, having a calming effect. Similarly Teas or Tinctures of Chamomile, Lemon Balm or Lemon Verbena Calm the Mind and Relieve Anxiety.

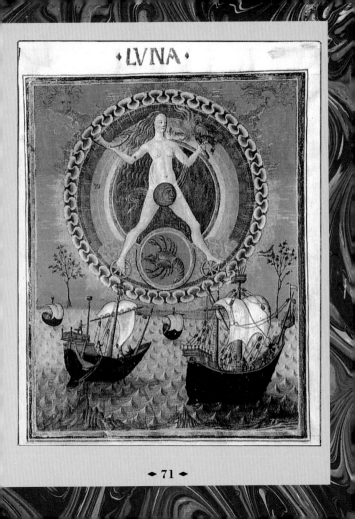

THE
HERBALL
OR GENERALL
Historie of
Plantes.

Gathered by John Gerarde
of London Master in
CHIRVRGERIE.

Imprinted at London by
Iohn Norton.
1597

A GALLIMAUFRY OF
HERBALIST'S DELIGHTS

There follows an **Interesting Selection** of **Receipts** gleaned from the writings of the **Great Herbalists**, each one bringing forth the true qualities of the Chosen Herb. Such Receipts provide Ample Quantities of the **Herb** employed for best **Medicinal Effect**. Many and Varied ideas are contained in these ancient receipts which can be adapted for the Modern Kitchen by cooks of Inspiration and Initiative.

John Nott's Candied Angelica

Boil the stalks of Angelica in water till they are tender; then peel them and put them in other warm water and cover them. Let them stand over a gentle fire till they become very green; then lay them on a cloth to dry; take their weight in Fine Sugar with a little Rose-water and boil it to a Candy height. Then put in your Angelica and boil them up quick; then take them for use.

Anthony Askham's Honey of Roses

Melrosette, or hony of roses is made thus; take faire purified hony and newe red roses . . . chop them small and boil togither . . . ye shall knowe by the sweet odour and the colour redde when it is boyled ynough.

Richard Pynsen's Tart of Borage Flowers

Take borage flowers and parboile them tender, then strayne them with the yolks of three or foure eggs and sweet curdes, or else take three or four apples and parboile with all, and strain them with sweete butter and a little mace . . . and so bake it.

Queen Henrietta Maria's Conserve of Borage

Take of fresh Borage flowers four ounces and of fine sugar twelve ounces, beat them well together in a stone Mortar and keep them in a vessel well glazed. This dish was created by the Queen's cook, known only as W.M.

Queen Henrietta Maria's Hyssop Syrup

Take a handful of Hyssop, of Figs, Raysins, Dates, of each an ounce, French Barley one ounce, boyl therein three pintes of fair water to a quart, strain and clarifye it with the Whytes of two Eggs, then put in two pound of fine Sugar and boyl it to a Syrop.

Another creation of W.M., as is the Receipt which follows.

Conserve of Flowers of Lavender

Take the flowers being new so many as you please, and beat them with three times their weight of fine White Sugar; they will keep one year. W.M. makes no suggestion as to the use, but a similar Receipt for Conserve of Rosemary is recommended as a relish with Game.

John Evelyn's Marigold Pudding

Take a pretty quantity of marygold flowers very well shred, mingle with a pint of cream on new milk and almost a pound of beef suet chop't very small, the gratings of a twopenny loaf and stirring all together put it into a bag flower'd and tie it fast. It will be boil'd within an hour or you might bake it in a pan.

Simple Comfrey Fritters

Make up a batter of egg flour and milk with a pinch of salt. Wash the Comfrey leaves and put them in the batter. Quickly fry until a golden brown.

Joseph Cooper's Pickled Cucumber in Dill

Gather the tops of the ripest Dill and cover the bottome of your vessel. Lay a layer of Cucumbers upon your Dill and then cover with another layer of the same. Proceed in this manner until you have fill'd your vessel to within a handful of the top. In as much water as you think will fill the vessel mix salt and allom to your taste and poure it upon them. Press them down with a stone.

The water will be best if boyl'd and cold which will keep it sweet. You may if it is your preference use a fine White Wine Vinegar in place of the allom.

Joseph Cooper was cook to Charles I.

A French Herbalist's Parsley Soup

Take milk, half its quantity of water, equal quantities of butter and flour together with one onion and a little salt. Melt the butter and to it add the flour, the liquids and the onion. Boil for one hour then remove the onion. Add cream to your and the yolk of two eggs. Warm carefully until the liquid has thickened. Before serving add a goodly amount of fresh finely chopped parsley.

John Evelyn's Tansie

Take the gratings or slices of three Naples-biscuits, put them into half a pint of cream, with twelve fresh eggs, four of the whites cast out, strain the rest and break them with two spoonsfull of rosewater, a little salt and sugar, half a grated nutmeg. And when ready for the pan, put almost a pint of juice of spinach, cleaver, beets, corn-sallet, green corn, violet or primrose tender leaves (for of any of these you may take your choice), with a very small sprig of tansie, and let it be fried so as to look green in the dish, with a strew of sugar, and store of the juice of orange. Some affect to have it fryed a little brown and crisp.

If this Receipt captures your attention for Adaptation in your kitchen, Take Heed of John Evelyn's careful use of Tansy. It should be used Very Sparingly. Even a sprig may prove an Excess for Modern Tastes.

John Evelyn's Pickled Nasturtium Buds

Gather the buds before they open to flower; lay them in the shade three or four hours and, putting them into an earthen glazed vessel, pour good vinegar on them and cover with a board. Thus let it stand for eight or ten days. Being taken out, and gently press'd, cast them into fresh vinegar and let them so remain as long as before. Repeat this a third time, and barrel them up with vinegar and a little salt. Some one hundred and fifty years later, in 1860, the estimable Mrs Beeton published a variation of this receipt which we print in later pages for your perusal.

And, Finally, to bring your Repast to a Slumberous End, enjoy a draught of

Queen Elizabeth's Hungary Water

Take one gallon brandy or clean spirits, to which add a handful each of Rosemary, Lavender and Myrtle, a handful being measured by cutting branches of the Herbs a goodly handspan in length. A Handful is the number of such branches which can be held in the hand. The said branches to be cut up into Half-finger Lengths and put to infuse the Brandy.

Queen Elizabeth of Hungary gave Her Assurance that this receipt provided the finest 'Hungary Water' 'twas possible to make.

CURE LIKE WITH LIKE

The Principles of Homeopathy were known to Ancient Greek Physicians such as Hippocrates in the Fifth Century BC. The very name of this Noble Healing Practice is derived from the Greek word *Homoios* which means 'like' and not, as is often Erroniously Thought from *Homo* meaning 'man'.

Homeopathy is the Art of Healing Like with Like. That is to say, Applying to an Illness a substance which produces Like Symptoms. Current Medical Opinion takes the view that Symptoms are a Direct Manifestation of the Illness. Homeopathy sees the Symptoms as the Reaction of the Body against the said Illness. Homeopathy seeks to Stimulate and not Supress this Reaction. Homeopathy is a Natural Healing Treatment, providing Remedies to Aid the Patient to regain health by Stimulating the Body's Natural Forces of Recovery.

Homeopathy treats the patient, rather than the disease

HOW HOMEOPATHY BEGAN

Known in Antiquity and practised through the Middle Ages and the Age of Enlightenment, the Homeopathic Principle *simila similibus curentur* 'let like be treated by like' often appears in *Materia Medica*. However, as practised in these times, Homeopathy derives from the work of Dr. Samuel Hahnemann, a German Physician at the Turn of the Eighteenth and Nineteenth Centuries.

Hahnemann found that Remedies obtained from Natural Materials, be they Animal, Vegetable or Mineral, were effective in Extreme Conditions. He experimented upon himself, administering small doses of Reputedly Poisonous Substances, taking note of the Symptoms

By Close Observation and Careful Experiment he established the Three Principles of Homeopathy

I A Medicine which in large doses produces the symptoms of a Disease will in small doses cure that disease.

II By Extreme Dilution, the medicine's Curative Properties are enhanced, and all the poisonous side effects are lost

III Homeopathic Remedies are Prescribed individually by the Study of the Whole Person, according to basic Temperament and Responses.

SELECTING YOUR REMEDY

Consulting a Homeopath is the Recommended Way to seek a Homeopathic Cure for your Ailment. However, it is possible to Treat Yourself by consulting Manuals of Homeopathy in Libraries or Emporia selling such cures.

I Consult the Index of Ailments to find the Medicines recommended for your Principal Symptoms

II Study the Description of the Medicines in the List of Medicines.

III Select the Medicine which Reflects your Total Symptoms, taking into account Appearance and Temperament.

For your Enlightenment, here is an Example of Diagnosis and Cure.

Consider a Young Lady, fair haired and blue eyed, of a Gentle, Emotional nature. She has had a Lingering and Unpleasant attack of Catarrh. Under Catarrh in an Index of Ailments she discovers that four Medicines are indicated for her Conditions viz: *Calc Fluor.*, *Euphrasia*, *Kali Bich.* and *Pulsatilla*. On consulting the Medicine Descriptions she will discover that *Pulsatilla* is the best medicine for her, suiting her Appearance and Temperament, the Nature of her Catarrhal Discharge and a Coincidence of Diet.

A Comprehensive List of Common Homepathic Medicines would be of No Purpose in this volume, but from a selection of their Common Names the Principle of using Poisons to Defeat Poisons is clear. In their Crudest Form they are a formidable Cabinet of Poisons. There is *Aconite* (the poisonous wolfsbane), *Arsenic* (most notorious poison of all), *Belladonna* (the deadly night-shade) and *Nux Vomica* (which produces strychine).

SELECTIVE INDEX OF AILMENTS
AND COMPLEMENTARY MEDICINES

Abdomen

Bloated after a light meal, with much flatulence; *Lycopodium* is recommended for those of Intense, Conscientious nature, unable to Endure Contradiction and Seek Argument.

Acne

For red-faced persons of a Cheerful Disposition, *Belladona*, for those of Fair Complexion, *Pulsatilla*,

Anxiety & Bereavement

Aconite is Effective in the Soothing of the Mind, Fear or Grief. For Prolonged Mourning, *Ignatia*, is suitable for Sensitive People who are easily moved to Tears.

Bad Breath

For a Bitter Taste on Waking, *Kalium Bichromiun* is suggested to Ease Mental Exertion which Exacerbates the Condition. A Metallic Taste and other Afflictions of the Mouth are treated with *Mercurius Solubilis*.

Boils

When there is Much Redness and Heat, *Belladonna* is effective when the Symptoms Worsen. When every Little Injury tends to Suppurate use *Silica*, particularly if of Light Complexion and Fine Skin.

Change of Life

Pulsatilla Relieves the Tensions for fair, blue-eyed women, whilst *Sepia* is efficacious for dark-haired women.

Chestiness

Bryonia relieves Dry Coughs, *Phosphorus* treats Hoarseness and Loss of Voice and *Sulphur* is best for those who Take Cold easily.

Chilblains

When Itchy and Swollen, take *Apis mellifica*, when Burning and Bluish-red, *Pulsatilla* provides relief.

Colds
Of sudden onset after Exposure to Draughts and Winds, *Aconite* provides Great Relief when Symptoms worsen at night, in inclement temperatures or while listening to music.

Constipation
The traditional aid to Effective Evacuation is *Nux Vomica*, whilst *Sulphur* can ease Difficult Passage.

Coughs
Dry Painful coughs respond well to *Bryonia*, whilst *Phosphorus* is efficaceous for treating hoarseness and Loss of Voice

Dandruff
Dry scaling scalps are best treated with *Graphites*.

Dyspepsia
Due to Excitement is calmed with *Argent. Nit.* whilst Flatulence in Chilly Persons who like fresh air is eased by *Carbo. veg.*

Fear
Following a frightening accident is assuaged by *Calc. Carb.* Of Crowds, Death or Impending Misfortune, *Ferr. Phos.* is recommended.

Hayfever

Burning, watering eyes are soothed by *Euphrasia*, but *Silica* is preferred for Chilly Individuals who suffer on waking.

Heartburn

Accompanied by stomach pain is eased by *Calc. Phos.*

Hot Flushes

Especially those of the face are cooled by *Graphites*, whilst excessive Perspiration is reduced by *Sepia*.

Insomnia

A Problem of Many Causes can variously be alleviated by *Aconite* for Much Twisting and Turning, *Arnica* for Simple Overtiredness and *Ignatia* for Compulsive Yawning.

Listlessness

For people of unsettled nature with an unnatural lack of activity, *Apis. mel.* is prescribed.

'Nerves'

Over-Anticipation of Coming Important Events can be calmed with *Argent. Nit.* whilst for a more Serious Inability to Cope with Life, *Gelsenium* should ease the Uncertainty.

Restlessness
For those with Acute Over-Imagination, *Aconite* is preferred, *Rhus. tox* being equally effective for those suffering from Night-time Apprehension.

Styes
Such Painful Afflications of the Eye Area can be eased at the onset with *Pulsatilla*, treated with *Graphites* if Discharging and *Phosporous* if producing a Burning Sensation.

Sunburn
Skin afflictions as a result of Over-exposure to the Rays of the Sun can be delayed by *Cantharides*; redness and heat are treated with *Belldonna*.

Toothache
For poor teeth *Calc. Fluor* can act as a Strengthener with *Calc. Carb* effective in reducing pain when exposed to Cold Air or Drink.

Travel Sickness
When caused by Restlessness and Nervousness, *Aconite* can soothe, when caused by the Movement of the Chosen Mode of Travel, *Nux. vom.* eases the Stomach.

Homeopathic Treatment for Ailments of Children.

A few Examples follow, but it is recommended that the Advice of Homeopathic Practitioners should be Sounded for Serious Problems.

Aconite is Good for the Child who catches Cold on Getting Wet and has Great Unsettled Sleep. *Arnica* soothes the Bumps and Bruises of Childhood and Shocks after some Little Mishap. *Arsen. Alb*. eases Tummy Pains, whilst *Belladonna* calms red skin and flushed faces after Great Excitments.

Pale-faced thin and lanky children are in need of *Calc. Phos, Drosera* is prescribed for Fits of Coughing and *Gelsenium* is a Remedy for Influenza. This latter Remedy is also a help for children who suffer from School Phobia and are Loathe to Attend their Place of Learning. Before important Examinations it can also help achieve a correct state of mind. The Over-Sensitive Child who easily Takes Offence benefits from *Hepar. Sulph*. and those of a Gentle, Yielding Disposition, given to Fear of Ghosts and the Dark and easily Moved to Tears are comforted by *Pulsatilla*. Excitable children, prone to Nosebleeds can be calmed with *Phosporous* and a Perspicacious Parent will administer *Nux. vom*. following Over-indulgence at Birthday Celebrations.

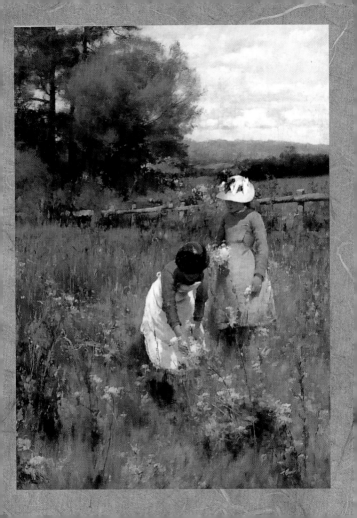

FENNEL SAUCE FOR MACKEREL.

412. INGREDIENTS.—½ pint of melted butter, No. 376, rather more than 1 tablespoonful of chopped fennel.

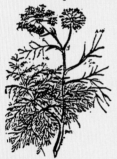

Mode.—Make the melted butter very smoothly, by recipe No. 376; chop the fennel rather small, carefully cleansing it from any grit or dirt, and put it to the butter when this is on the point of boiling. Simmer for a minute or two, and serve in a tureen.

Time.—2 minutes. *Average cost,* 4d.

Sufficient to serve with 5 or 6 mackerel.

SEED BISCUITS.

1749. INGREDIENTS.—1 lb. of flour, ¼ lb. of sifted sugar, ¼ lb. of butter, ½ oz. of caraway seeds, 3 eggs.

Mode.—Beat the butter to a cream; stir in the flour, sugar, and caraway seeds; and when these ingredients are well mixed, add the eggs, which should be well whisked. Roll out the paste, with a round cutter shape out the biscuits, and bake them in a moderate oven from 10 to 15 minutes. The tops of the biscuits may be brushed over with a little milk or the white of an egg, and then a little sugar strewn over.

Time.—10 to 15 minutes. *Average cost,* 1s.

Sufficient to make 3 dozen biscuits. *Seasonable* at any time.

PICKLED NASTURTIUMS (a very good Substitute for Capers)

482. INGREDIENTS.—To each pint of vinegar, 1 oz. of salt, 6 pepper-corns, nasturtiums.

Mode.—Gather the nasturtium-pods on a dry day, and wipe them clean with a cloth; put them in a dry glass bottle, with vinegar, salt, and pepper in the above proportion. If you cannot find enough ripe to fill a bottle, cork up what you have got until you have some more fit: they may be added from day to day. Bung up the bottles, and seal or rosin the tops. They will be fit for use in 10 or 12 months; and the best way is to make them one season for the next.

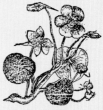

NASTURTIUMS.

Seasonable.—Look for nasturtium-pods from the end of July to the end of August.

PARSLEY JUICE, for Colouring various Dishes.

495. Procure some nice young parsley; wash it and dry it thoroughly in a cloth; pound the leaves in a mortar till all the juice is extracted, and put the juice in a teacup or small jar; place this in a saucepan of boiling water, and warm it on the *bain marie* principle just long enough to take off its rawness; let it drain, and it will be ready for colouring.

TO PRESERVE PARSLEY THROUGH THE WINTER.

496. Use freshly-gathered parsley for keeping, and wash it perfectly free from grit and dirt; put it into boiling water which has been slightly salted and well skimmed, and then let it boil for 2 or 3 minutes; take it out, let it drain, and lay it on a sieve in front of the fire, when it should be dried as expeditiously as possible. Store it away in a very dry place in bottles, and when wanted for use, pour over it a little warm water, and let it stand for about 5 minutes.

Seasonable.—This may be done at any time between June and October.

YOUR HERB KITCHEN

Herbs can be added to almost every Receipt in Quantities to suit your taste. While they can add a little touch of Extra Flavour or Aroma, there are many Receipts in which the Herb is a More Important Ingredient, thus ensuring that you have a sufficiency to Benefit from their Therapeutic effect.

Coriander

The Seeds and Leaves of Coriander are Good for the Digestion and are much used in Dishes from Araby and the East. The Seeds have a Stronger Effect and Ease Abdominal Cramps and Promote Ease of Digestion. The Leaves have a similar, but weaker, Effect. What better way to Ingest goodly quantities than to Partake of **Chicken with Two Corianders**.

Take breast pieces from a Chicken which has enjoyed the freedom of the Barnyard. Cut into thin strips and allow to lie in Lemon Juice for two hours or more. Finely slice some Red Peppers, a modicum of fresh Ginger and Garlic. In a Stirring Pan heat some Groundnut Oil until it smokes. Reduce heat and throw in the peppers, ginger and garlic, together with two teaspoons of Ground Coriander Seeds. After a moment stir in the chicken slices and cook quickly for but a few moments more.

Add the Lemon Juice previously employed, together with Condiments to your taste. Stir in a goodly handful of fresh Coriander Leaves and Serve with Haste.

Basil

The Aromatic Leaves of Basil are good for the Brain, clearing the Head and Sharpening the Memory. In the Countries of the Levant,people eat much of Basil in the evenings to promote Sleep and drink an Infusion of it in the Morn to bring Alertness. **Potato Salad with Red Basil Paste & Fresh Basil** provides an Amplitude of the herb. Make a paste of Basil Leaves, ground with Olive Oil, Garlic, Nuts from the Pine and Tomatoes Dried in the Sun. Boil Fine New Potatoes, drain and allow to cool. Anoint with the Basil Paste. Tear apart the plentiful numbers of fresh basil leaves and strew over the salad.

Bulthe Baſill, oz ſmall Baſill gentle.

Parsley

The Tonic Qualities of Parsley have been Fully Documented in these pages and Fulsome Quantities in Salads and as Garnishes are always to be advised. A more Robust Dish for Chilly Winter is **Parsley Dumplings**. Traditional Dumplings contain Suet, which unfortunately Render this Dish unsuitable for Vegetarians. The suet must be finely grated and chopped before use. To sifted Flour add half its weight of Shredded Suet, a sprinkling of Salt and goodly amounts of Chopped Parsley. Knead well. Roll the mixture into egg-sized balls. Bring a deep pan of Stock or Broth to the boil. Gently immerse the dumplings and simmer until ready.

Thyme

For stimulation of the Heart and Inducing a good Antiseptic into the System, Thyme is the Ideal Herb. Its Aromatic Qualities blend perfectly with the Smokiness of a good cured Bacon in another Winter Dish, **Thyme and Bacon Dumplings**. Dice the Smoked Bacon and one small Onion. Fry the bacon in a little butter, add the onion and a few small sprigs of Thyme. When Soft and Golden, season to your taste and add to a Dumpling mixture and cook in the mode employed for **Parsley Dumplings**.

Fennel

Its Aniseed flavour and Crispy Crunchiness make it useful for Salads. For an Ample Filling, but not Fattening Dish what could be better than **Fennel Bulb with Fennel Seeds**. Take sufficient for your needs of Fennel Bulbs. Trim and slice, first in half and then downwards into Substantial Segments. Heat some Good Olive Oil in a Pan for Frying, add the Fennel pieces, together with a good teaspoonful of Fennel Seeds. Stir vigorously for a few moments, cover and cook until the pieces brown slightly. Season with Salt from the Sea and Freshly Ground Black Pepper.

Sage

So powerful was it thought to be in Medieval Times that it was said 'Why dieth the man in whose garden Sage grows'. Sage has a strong Resinous Flavour so should be used Sparingly in receipts such as **Savoury Sage Stuffing**, a versatile dish which can be used to Fill such Vegetables as Diverse as Mushrooms and Courgettes. Bind together with one ounce of butter, a little chopped Onion, Wholewheat Breadcrumbs, a little each of Thyme and Marjoram, Seasoning to your taste and a larger amount of Dried Sage. A little water may be added to moisten the mixture. Use this to fill your Favourite Vegetable or Bird before Baking or Roasting.

HEAVENLY HEALING HERBS

Nicholas Culpeper, though Revered as a Herbalist, was much Critized for his conviction that there was a close relationship between Astrology and the Efficacy of Herbal Preparations. In his *Herbal,* the Signs of the Zodiac had a Dual Purpose: they influenced the growing and collecting of plants and were identified with the various parts of the Human Body they governed.

HERBS AND THEIR PLANETS

Agrimoney – Jupiter	Marjoram – Mercury
Balm – Jupiter	Mints – Venus
Basil – Mars	Mugwort – Venus
Bay – Sun	Oregano – Mercury
Borage – Jupiter	Parsley – Mercury
Caraway – Mercury	Pennyroyal – Venus
Catnip – Venus	Rosemary – Sun
Chamomile – Sun	Rue – Sun
Chives – Mars	Sage – Jupiter
Dill – Mercury	Savory – Mercury
Fennel – Mercury	Tarrgon – Mars
Hyssop – Jupiter	Wormwood – Mars
Lavender – Mercury	Yarrow – Venus

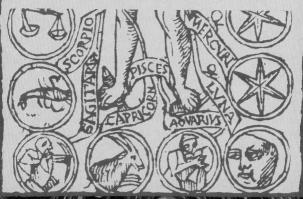

Jupiter rules the thighs and liver; Mars rules the head, pelvis and sex organs; the Sun rules the heart and spine; Mercury rules the arms and lungs and Venus rules the kidneys and the lower back. And so the most efficaceous Herbal Remedy will be found amongst those under the Governance of an appropriate planet.

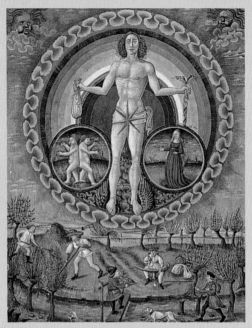

'The admirable Harmony of the Creation is herein seen, in the influence of Stars up on Herbs and the Body of Man, how one part of the Creation is subservient to another, and all for the use of Man'
Nicholas Culpeper